I0830304

Braving Breast Cancer

Finding Inner Strength and Overcoming Adversity

by

ALANNA MCKINNEY

Copyright © by ALANNA MCKINNEY 2022. All rights reserved.

Before this document is duplicated or reproduced in any manner, the publisher's consent must be gained. Therefore, the contents within can neither be stored electronically, transferred, nor kept in a database. Neither in Part nor full can the document be copied, scanned, faxed, or retained without approval from the publisher or creator.

Contents

Introduction
Overview of Breast Cancer

Breast cancer is a type of cancer that begins in the cells of the breast. It is the most common cancer among women worldwide, and affects both men and women, although it is less common in men. The breast is composed of glandular and fatty tissue, and when cancer cells form in the glandular tissue, it is called ductal carcinoma. If the cancer cells form in the fatty tissue, it is called lobular carcinoma.

Breast cancer occurs when abnormal cells in the breast grow and divide in an uncontrolled way. These abnormal cells can form a tumor, which can be benign (not cancerous) or malignant (cancerous). If left untreated, malignant tumors can grow, invade nearby tissues, and spread to other parts of the body through the bloodstream or lymphatic system.

Risk factors for developing breast cancer include age, gender, genetics, family history, hormonal factors (such as starting menstruation early or entering menopause late), exposure to radiation, alcohol consumption, and obesity. There is also evidence that certain lifestyle factors, such as diet and physical activity, can play a role in the development of breast cancer.

Early detection is key to successful treatment and recovery from breast cancer. Women should perform monthly self-exams and have regular mammograms to screen for breast cancer. Other screening methods include clinical breast exams and

MRI scans. If a breast abnormality is detected, a biopsy may be performed to determine if the cells are cancerous.

Treatment for breast cancer depends on the type and stage of cancer, as well as the patient's overall health and personal preferences. Treatment options include surgery, radiation therapy, chemotherapy, hormone therapy, and targeted therapy. In some cases, a combination of these treatments may be recommended.

It is important to remember that breast cancer is a highly treatable disease, and many people with breast cancer go on to live full and healthy lives after treatment. With advances in technology and medicine, there are more options available than ever before for those facing a breast cancer diagnosis. Seeking the support of family, friends, and a medical team can also be crucial in navigating the physical and emotional challenges of breast cancer.

The Importance of Early Detection and Treatment

Early detection and treatment of breast cancer are crucial in improving outcomes and increasing the chances of a successful recovery. Early detection allows for treatment to begin when the cancer is still in its earliest stages when it is often most treatable. In contrast, waiting until cancer has progressed can result in a poorer prognosis and more limited treatment options.

Mammograms are the most commonly used screening tool for breast cancer and are recommended for women over the age of 40. Women with a higher risk of developing breast cancer, such as those with a strong family history or a genetic predisposition, may need to start getting mammograms at an earlier age. Clinical breast exams and MRI scans can also be used to detect breast cancer.

Self-exams are also an important part of early detection, as they allow women to become familiar with their bodies and detect any changes or abnormalities. Women should perform self-exams regularly, such as once a month, to check for any changes in their breasts.

If breast cancer is detected early, treatment options may include surgery, radiation therapy, chemotherapy, hormone therapy, and targeted therapy. In some cases, a combination of these treatments may be recommended. Early detection also allows for a better chance of breast conservation, where only the cancerous tissue is removed and the rest of the breast is preserved.

Treating breast cancer in its early stages also increases the chances of avoiding more extensive and invasive treatments, such as mastectomy or extensive radiation therapy. It can also reduce the risk of cancer spreading to other parts of the body, which can result in a poorer prognosis and a lower quality of life.

In addition to improving outcomes, early detection and treatment of breast cancer can also be a crucial factor in reducing the cost and burden of care. Early treatment can help to avoid more expensive and time-consuming treatments, such as multiple surgeries or prolonged hospital stays.

In conclusion, early detection and treatment of breast cancer are essential for improving outcomes and increasing the chances of a successful recovery. Regular mammograms, self-exams, and working closely with a healthcare team can all play a crucial role in the early detection and treatment of breast cancer.

CHAPTER 1
Understanding Your Diagnosis

Receiving a diagnosis of breast cancer can be a confusing and overwhelming experience. It is important to take the time to understand your diagnosis so that you can make informed decisions about your care and treatment.

The first step in understanding your diagnosis is to gather information about your specific type of breast cancer. This may include information about the size of the tumor, the stage of cancer, and whether it has spread to other parts of the body. This information will help you and your healthcare team determine the best course of treatment.

It is also important to understand the different types of treatment options available. These may include surgery, radiation therapy, chemotherapy, hormone therapy, and targeted therapy. Each type of treatment has its benefits and risks, and your healthcare team can help you weigh the options to determine the best treatment plan for you.

Another important aspect of understanding your diagnosis is to understand the potential side effects of treatment. These may include physical side effects, such as fatigue, nausea, and hair loss, as well as emotional side effects, such as depression and anxiety. Understanding these potential side effects can help you prepare for the treatment process and make arrangements for support during your recovery.

It is also important to understand the importance of following up with your healthcare team after treatment. This may include regular mammograms, clinical breast exams, and doctor visits to monitor your health and check for any signs of recurrence.

It is also important to seek support during this time. This may include talking to family and friends, joining a support group, or seeking counseling. Having a support system can help you navigate the emotional challenges of a breast cancer diagnosis and provide you with a source of encouragement and support.

Understanding your breast cancer diagnosis is an important step in the journey toward recovery. By taking the time to gather information, understand your treatment options, prepare for side effects, and seek support, you can take control of your care and improve your chances of a successful outcome.

Also, receiving a diagnosis of breast cancer can be a life-changing experience. However, by taking the time to understand your diagnosis and treatment options, you can increase your chances of a successful recovery.

One of the first steps in understanding your diagnosis is to gather information about your specific type of breast cancer. This may include information about the size of the tumor, the stage of cancer, and whether it has spread to other parts of the body. This information will help you and your healthcare team determine the best course of treatment.

It is also important to understand the different types of treatment options available. These may include:

1. **Surgery**: Surgery is one of the most common treatments for breast cancer. It may involve a lumpectomy, which removes the cancerous tissue and a small amount of surrounding tissue, or a mastectomy, which removes the entire breast. In some cases, reconstruction surgery may be performed to restore the shape of the breast.

2. **Radiation therapy**: Radiation therapy uses high-energy radiation to kill cancer cells and shrink tumors. This treatment is typically given after surgery and may be recommended for certain types of breast cancer.

3. **Chemotherapy**: Chemotherapy uses drugs to kill cancer cells and shrink tumors. This treatment may be given before or after surgery and may be recommended for certain types of breast cancer.

4. **Hormone therapy**: Hormone therapy is used to treat breast cancers that are fueled by hormones, such as estrogen. This treatment may involve taking hormone-blocking drugs or having surgery to remove the ovaries.

5. **Targeted therapy**: Targeted therapy is a type of treatment that uses drugs to target specific genes or proteins that are involved in the growth of cancer cells. This type of therapy may be recommended for certain types of breast cancer.

It is important to understand the potential side effects of each type of treatment so that you can make informed decisions about your care and treatment. These may include physical side effects, such as fatigue, nausea, and hair loss, as well as emotional side effects, such as depression and anxiety. Your healthcare team can provide you with more information about the side effects of each type of treatment and help you prepare for the treatment process.

It is also important to understand the importance of following up with your healthcare team after treatment. This may include regular mammograms, clinical breast exams, and doctor visits to monitor your health and check for any signs of recurrence.

Finally, seeking support is an important part of the recovery process. This may include talking to family and friends, joining a support group, or seeking counseling. Having a support system can help you navigate the emotional challenges of a breast cancer diagnosis and provide you with a source of encouragement and support.

In conclusion, understanding your breast cancer diagnosis is an important step in the journey toward recovery. By gathering information, understanding your treatment options, preparing for side effects, following up with your healthcare team, and seeking support, you can take control of your care and increase your chances of a successful outcome.

The Stages of Breast Cancer

Breast cancer is a disease that occurs when abnormal cells in the breast divide and grow without control. The stage of breast cancer refers to the extent to which cancer has spread within the breast or to other parts of the body. Understanding the stages of breast cancer can help you and your healthcare team determine the best course of treatment and predict the outcome of the disease.

There are four main stages of breast cancer, as follows:

1. **Stage 0**: In stage 0, the cancer is confined to the ducts within the breast and has not spread to other parts of the body. This stage is also known as ductal carcinoma in situ (DCIS).

2. **Stage I**: In stage I, the cancer is still confined to the breast, but is larger than in stage 0. The size of the tumor may be up to 2 centimeters, and cancer may have spread to the lymph nodes near the breast.

3. **Stage II**: In stage II, cancer may have grown larger than 2 centimeters, or has spread to more lymph nodes near the breast. Cancer may also have spread to the nearby chest wall or skin, but has not spread to other parts of the body.

4. **Stage III**: In stage III, cancer has spread beyond the breast and nearby lymph nodes to other parts of the body, such as the bones, liver, lungs, or brain. This stage is also known as advanced breast cancer.

Staging is an important part of the diagnostic process, as it helps determine the appropriate course of treatment. The treatment options for each stage of breast cancer may vary and may include surgery, radiation therapy, chemotherapy, hormone therapy, and targeted therapy.

It is also important to understand that there is no single standard treatment for each stage of breast cancer. Your healthcare team will take into consideration a variety of factors, including the size and location of the tumor, the type of breast cancer, and your overall health, when determining the best course of treatment.

In addition to traditional treatments, there are also alternative and complementary therapies that may help relieve symptoms and improve the quality of life for those with breast cancer. These may include massage therapy, acupuncture, and nutritional therapy, among others.

It is important to remember that a breast cancer diagnosis is not a death sentence and that many people with breast cancer can successfully manage the disease and return to a healthy and fulfilling life. By understanding the stages of breast cancer and working closely with your healthcare team, you can increase your chances of a successful outcome.

Types of Treatment Options

Breast cancer treatment options vary depending on the stage and type of breast cancer, as well as the individual's overall health and personal preferences. In general, the most common treatment options for breast cancer include surgery, radiation therapy, chemotherapy, hormone therapy, and targeted therapy. Some individuals may also choose to undergo alternative and complementary therapies to relieve symptoms and improve their quality of life.

. **Surgery**: Surgery is the most common treatment for breast cancer, and several types of surgical procedures may be used, including:

- **Lumpectomy**: Also known as breast-conserving surgery, a lumpectomy removes the cancerous tissue and a small amount of surrounding healthy tissue.

- **Mastectomy**: A mastectomy is a procedure in which the entire breast is removed. There are several types of mastectomy procedures, including total mastectomy, modified radical mastectomy, and radical mastectomy.

- **Sentinel lymph node biopsy**: This is a procedure in which a small number of the lymph nodes closest to the breast are removed and examined for cancer cells.

2. **Radiation Therapy**: Radiation therapy uses high-energy beams, such as X-rays, to kill cancer cells. This treatment is often used after surgery to help reduce the risk of cancer recurrence. Radiation therapy may also be used as the primary treatment for early-stage breast cancer or for individuals who are unable to undergo surgery.

3. **Chemotherapy**: Chemotherapy is a type of cancer treatment that uses drugs to kill cancer cells. This treatment is usually given in cycles, with periods of treatment followed by periods of rest. Chemotherapy may be used in combination with surgery or radiation therapy, or as a standalone treatment for advanced-stage breast cancer.

4. **Hormone Therapy**: Hormone therapy is a type of treatment that targets hormones, such as estrogen, which can fuel the growth of certain types of breast cancer cells. Hormone therapy

may be used as the primary treatment for hormone-receptor-positive breast cancer, or as a complementary treatment to help reduce the risk of cancer recurrence.

5. **Targeted Therapy**: Targeted therapy is a type of treatment that targets specific proteins or genetic changes within cancer cells. This type of treatment is often used in combination with other treatments, such as chemotherapy, to help improve treatment outcomes.

In addition to traditional treatments, there are also alternative and complementary therapies that may help relieve symptoms and improve the quality of life for those with breast cancer. These may include massage therapy, acupuncture, and nutritional therapy, among others.

It is important to work closely with your healthcare team to determine the best course of treatment for your individual needs. This may involve considering a variety of factors, including the stage and type of breast cancer, your overall health, and your personal preferences. With the right treatment plan, many individuals with breast cancer can successfully manage the disease and return to a healthy and fulfilling life.

Working with Your Healthcare Team

Working with your healthcare team is an essential component of managing breast cancer. Your healthcare team will typically include a variety of medical professionals, including:

1. **Surgeon**: A surgeon is typically the first medical professional you will see after a breast cancer diagnosis. They can perform a biopsy to confirm the diagnosis and help determine the best surgical options for your case.

2. **Medical Oncologist**: A medical oncologist is a doctor who specializes in treating cancer with medication. They may recommend chemotherapy, hormone therapy, or targeted therapy to treat breast cancer.

3. **Radiation Oncologist**: A radiation oncologist is a doctor who specializes in using radiation therapy to treat cancer. They may recommend radiation therapy as part of your breast cancer treatment plan.

4. **Radiologist**: A radiologist is a doctor who specializes in interpreting imaging tests, such as mammograms and MRI scans. They can help determine the size, location, and extent of your breast cancer.

5. **Pathologist**: A pathologist is a doctor who specializes in diagnosing diseases by analyzing tissue samples. They will examine your biopsy samples to determine the type and stage of your breast cancer.

In addition to these medical professionals, your healthcare team may also include a variety of other healthcare professionals, such as nurse practitioners, physician assistants, nurses, and dietitians.

It is important to have open and honest communication with your healthcare team. This includes sharing any concerns or questions you may have and keeping them informed of any changes in your symptoms or overall health. Your healthcare team can help you understand your diagnosis and treatment options, and provide support and resources to help you manage the physical and emotional effects of breast cancer.

It can also be helpful to have a support system in place, such as family, friends, or support groups. This can provide a source of emotional support and help you feel less isolated during what can be a challenging time.

Overall, working with your healthcare team and having a strong support system in place can help you navigate the physical, emotional, and practical aspects of managing breast cancer. With the right support and resources, many individuals can successfully manage their diagnosis and maintain a high quality of life.

It is also important to keep a record of your medical history and treatment plan, including any medications you are taking, test results, and appointments. This can help ensure that all members of your healthcare team are on the same page, and that important information is not lost or overlooked.

It may also be helpful to consider a second opinion, especially if you are unsure about your diagnosis or treatment plan. A second opinion can help you understand the available options and make informed decisions about your care.

Another important aspect of working with your healthcare team is managing treatment-related side effects. Many treatments for breast cancer can cause physical and emotional side effects, such as fatigue, pain, nausea, hair loss, and changes in skin, nails, and bones. Your healthcare team can provide strategies to help manage these side effects and improve your overall quality of life.

It is also important to understand that breast cancer treatment is a highly individualized process, and what works for one person may not work for another. Your healthcare team can help you understand the available options and develop a treatment plan that meets your unique needs and goals.

Finally, it is important to maintain open communication with your healthcare team, even after treatment is completed. Regular follow-up appointments and ongoing monitoring can help detect any recurrence or new developments, and ensure that any necessary interventions are taken on time.

Working with your healthcare team is an ongoing process, and it is important to have the right support and resources in place to help you manage your diagnosis and treatment. With the right care and support, many individuals with breast cancer can successfully manage the disease and maintain a high quality of life.

CHAPTER 2

Coping with Emotional Challenges

Breast cancer can be a challenging and overwhelming experience, both physically and emotionally. It is common for individuals to experience a wide range of emotions, such as fear, anger, sadness, and anxiety. It is important to understand that these emotions are normal and that there are resources and strategies available to help manage them.

One important aspect of coping with the emotional challenges of breast cancer is building a strong support system. This can include friends, family, support groups, or counseling services. Talking to someone who understands what you are going through can help reduce feelings of isolation and provide a source of emotional support.

It can also be helpful to educate yourself about breast cancer and the different treatment options. Having a better understanding of what to expect can help reduce feelings of uncertainty and fear.

Another important aspect of coping with the emotional challenges of breast cancer is finding healthy ways to manage stress. This can include engaging in physical activity, such as yoga or exercise, practicing relaxation techniques, such as deep breathing or meditation, or engaging in creative activities, such as painting or writing.

t is also important to maintain a healthy lifestyle, including
eating a well-balanced diet, getting enough sleep, and avoiding
harmful behaviors, such as smoking and excessive alcohol
consumption.

t may also be helpful to seek professional counseling or
therapy. A counselor or therapist can help you process your
emotions and provide support and coping strategies to help
manage the physical and emotional effects of breast cancer.

t is important to understand that the emotional challenges of
breast cancer can be ongoing and may persist even after
treatment is completed. It is important to continue seeking
support and finding healthy ways to manage stress to maintain
your overall well-being.

Coping with the emotional challenges of breast cancer is a
journey that requires time, patience, and the right support. With
the right resources and strategies in place, many individuals
can successfully manage the physical and emotional effects of
breast cancer and maintain a high quality of life.

Additionally, it may also be helpful to participate in support
groups, either in person or online. Support groups can provide
a safe and supportive environment where you can connect with
others who are going through similar experiences and share
your feelings, thoughts, and concerns. You can also learn
about the latest treatments and resources available, as well as
gain valuable advice and support from others who have gone
through the same process.

Another important aspect of coping with the emotional challenges of breast cancer is practicing self-care. This can include setting boundaries, taking time for yourself, and engaging in activities that bring you joy and relaxation. It can also be helpful to prioritize your physical and mental health and make sure that you are taking care of yourself in ways that are meaningful to you.

It is also important to be proactive in managing any symptoms of depression, anxiety, or other mental health conditions that may arise during and after treatment. If you are feeling overwhelmed, it is important to seek help from your healthcare team or a mental health professional. They can provide you with resources and strategies to help manage these symptoms and improve your overall well-being.

Finally, it is important to understand that the emotional impact of breast cancer can be different for everyone. There is no right or wrong way to feel, and everyone's journey is unique. It is important to find the right support and resources that work for you and to be patient and compassionate with yourself as you navigate the emotional ups and downs of the breast cancer journey.

In conclusion, coping with the emotional challenges of breast cancer requires time, patience, and the right support. With the right resources and strategies in place, many individuals can successfully manage the emotional impact of the disease and maintain a high quality of life. Remember that it is okay to reach out for help and support and that there are many resources available to help you along the way.

Dealing with Fear and Anxiety

Fear and anxiety are normal emotions to experience when facing a breast cancer diagnosis. The uncertainty, potential physical changes, and fear of recurrence can be overwhelming. However, it is possible to manage these feelings and reduce their impact on your life.

One important aspect of dealing with fear and anxiety is educating yourself about breast cancer and the different treatment options. This can help reduce feelings of uncertainty and empower you to make informed decisions about your care.

It is also important to build a strong support system. This can include friends, family, support groups, or counseling services. Talking to someone who understands what you are going through can help reduce feelings of isolation and provide a source of emotional support.

Another important aspect of dealing with fear and anxiety is finding healthy ways to manage stress. This can include engaging in physical activity, such as yoga or exercise, practicing relaxation techniques, such as deep breathing or meditation, or engaging in creative activities, such as painting or writing.

It is also important to maintain a healthy lifestyle, including eating a well-balanced diet, getting enough sleep, and avoiding harmful behaviors, such as smoking and excessive alcohol consumption.

Cognitive-behavioral therapy (CBT) can also be effective in reducing fear and anxiety. CBT is a type of therapy that focuses on the thoughts and beliefs that contribute to negative emotions and helps individuals develop new, more positive patterns of thinking.

Additionally, medication may be an option for individuals who are struggling with severe anxiety or depression. Antidepressants and anti-anxiety medications can help reduce symptoms and improve overall well-being.

It is important to understand that fear and anxiety can be ongoing and may persist even after treatment is completed. It is important to continue seeking support and finding healthy ways to manage stress to maintain your overall well-being.

In conclusion, dealing with fear and anxiety is a journey that requires time, patience, and the right support. With the right resources and strategies in place, many individuals can successfully manage the emotional impact of breast cancer and maintain a high quality of life. It is important to remember that it is okay to reach out for help and support and that there are many resources available to help you along the way.

In addition to the strategies mentioned above, there are several other ways to cope with fear and anxiety related to breast cancer. These include:

1. **Mindfulness and relaxation techniques**: Practicing mindfulness can help reduce anxiety and improve overall well-being. This can include engaging in mindfulness-based stress reduction (MBSR), progressive muscle relaxation, guided imagery, or other forms of meditation.

2. **Exercise**: Regular physical activity can help improve mood and reduce anxiety. Exercise can also help improve physical health and boost overall energy levels.

3. **Support groups**: Joining a support group for individuals facing similar experiences can be a great source of emotional support and can help reduce feelings of isolation and loneliness.

4. **Talk therapy**: Talking with a mental health professional, such as a psychologist or counselor, can help you process your feelings and develop coping strategies.

5. **Art therapy**: Engaging in creative activities, such as painting or drawing, can be a therapeutic way to express emotions and reduce anxiety.

6. **Journaling**: Writing down your thoughts and feelings can help you process and understand your emotions, and can also serve as a valuable source of support.

7. **Meditation and yoga**: These practices can help reduce stress and improve overall well-being, both physically and emotionally.

8. **Spending time in nature**: Engaging in activities such as hiking, gardening, or bird watching can help reduce stress and improve overall well-being.

9. **Seek support from loved ones**: Sharing your thoughts and feelings with friends, family, or a trusted support person can help you feel heard and supported.

It is important to find the strategies that work best for you and to be patient with yourself as you work through your emotions. It is also important to understand that fear and anxiety can be ongoing and may persist even after treatment is completed and that it is okay to seek support at any time.

In conclusion, dealing with fear and anxiety related to breast cancer can be challenging, but there are many resources and strategies available to help you manage these emotions. With the right support, it is possible to maintain a high quality of life and feel empowered in your journey toward recovery.

Building a Support System

Building a strong support system is an important part of the breast cancer journey. Having people in your life who are there for you can provide you with comfort, encouragement, and a sense of community as you navigate through this experience.

Here are some tips for building a support system:

1. **Reach out to friends and family**: Let your loved ones know how they can help and what you need from them. Whether it's a phone call, a visit, or just a text to let you know they are thinking of you, your friends and family can be a valuable source of support.

2. **Connect with other breast cancer survivors**: Joining a breast cancer support group can provide you with a sense of community and the opportunity to connect with others who understand what you're going through.

3. Consider joining an online support group: Many online communities are available that provide support and resources for those facing breast cancer. These can be great resources for connecting with others who are experiencing similar challenges and for finding information and resources.

4. **Find a support person who is knowledgeable about breast cancer**: Having someone knowledgeable about breast cancer, such as a doctor, nurse, or social worker, can help answer questions and provide support and guidance.

5. **Consider hiring a professional caregiver**: Hiring a professional caregiver can provide you with additional support and help alleviate stress, allowing you to focus on your health and well-being.

6. **Seek support from your religious or spiritual community**: Many religious and spiritual communities

offer support groups and other resources for those facing cancer.

7. **Take advantage of community resources**: Many communities offer resources such as free transportation, meals, and financial assistance for those facing breast cancer.

Having a strong support system can make a significant difference in your experience with breast cancer. It is important to be proactive in seeking out support and to be open and honest about your needs and feelings. Your support system can provide you with comfort, encouragement, and a sense of community as you navigate through this experience, and help you feel empowered and resilient as you work toward recovery.

In addition to the tips mentioned earlier, here are some additional ways to build and strengthen your support system:

1. **Seek support from a counselor or therapist**: Talking to a mental health professional can help manage your emotions and cope with the challenges of breast cancer. They can help you develop coping strategies and provide a safe space for you to express your feelings.

2. **Get involved in a hobby or activity**: Joining a club or participating in a hobby can provide you with a sense of purpose, help you forget about your worries for a while, and provide a sense of community.

3. **Focus on self-care**: Taking care of yourself is essential during the breast cancer journey. Whether it's through exercise, meditation, or other activities that help you relax and recharge, self-care can provide an escape from stress and improve your overall well-being.

4. **Build a network of medical support**: Building a network of healthcare professionals who are familiar with your case can provide you with a sense of security and help ensure that your needs are being met.

5. **Lean on your partner**: If you have a partner, they can be a valuable source of support during your breast cancer journey. Encourage them to be involved in your care and provide them with the information and resources they need to support you.

6. **Connect with organizations that support those with breast cancer**: There are many organizations and foundations dedicated to supporting those with breast cancer. Connecting with these organizations can provide you with information, resources, and a sense of community.

7. **Celebrate your successes**: Celebrating your successes, no matter how small, can provide you with a sense of accomplishment and help you maintain a positive outlook.

Having a strong support system can help you cope with the physical, emotional, and practical challenges of breast cancer. Building and strengthening your support system is a process, and it is important to reach out for help when you need it. With the right support and resources, you can navigate the breast cancer journey with confidence and resilience.

Finding Ways to Cope and Stay Positive

Dealing with a diagnosis of breast cancer can be overwhelming and can take an emotional toll. However, it is important to find ways to cope and stay positive during the breast cancer journey. Here are some strategies that can help:

Focus on what you can control: While it can be difficult, try to focus on what you can control, such as your attitude, outlook, and approach to treatment. This can help you feel more in control and reduce feelings of helplessness.

Practice gratitude: Cultivating an attitude of gratitude can help shift your focus away from what you're struggling with and instead focus on what you're thankful for. This can be as simple as keeping a gratitude journal or making a daily list of things you're grateful for.

Connect with others: Connecting with others who have been through a similar experience can provide a sense of community and comfort. Joining a support group or online community can provide you with a safe and supportive space to connect with others who understand what you're going through.

Stay active: Regular physical activity, such as walking or yoga, can improve your mood and reduce stress. Exercise also has physical health benefits, which can be especially important during treatment.

Practice self-care: Taking care of yourself is crucial during the breast cancer journey. This can include activities like getting enough sleep, eating a healthy diet, and engaging in stress-reducing activities like meditation or massage.

Get creative: Engaging in creative activities, such as painting or writing, can be a great way to express yourself and process your emotions.

Seek professional help: If you're struggling with emotional or psychological challenges, consider seeking the help of a mental health professional. Talking to a counselor or therapist can provide you with the support and resources you need to cope with the emotional challenges of breast cancer.

Stay positive: Maintaining a positive outlook can be difficult, but it can also be incredibly empowering. Surround yourself with positive people, focus on what you're grateful for, and find ways to maintain a positive outlook even in tough times.

Everyone copes with breast cancer in their way, and what works for one person may not work for another. The important thing is to find what works for you and to reach out for help when you need it. With the right support and resources, you can navigate the breast cancer journey with resilience and positivity.

CHAPTER 3

Navigating the Physical Challenges

Dealing with the physical challenges of breast cancer can be difficult, but there are ways to manage the symptoms and improve your quality of life. Here are some strategies to help you navigate the physical challenges:

- **Stay informed**: Educate yourself about the physical side effects of your treatment, such as fatigue, pain, or changes in skin or hair. Understanding what to expect can help you prepare and take steps to manage these symptoms.

- **Manage side effects**: If you're experiencing side effects from your treatment, talk to your healthcare team about ways to manage them. They may be able to provide medication, advice, or other strategies to help relieve symptoms.

- **Stay active**: Regular physical activity can help boost your energy, improve your mood, and promote physical healing. It's important to find an activity that you enjoy and that you can stick to, even during treatment.

- **Eat well**: Eating a balanced diet that's rich in nutrients can help you feel better and support your overall health during treatment. Talk to your healthcare team about what types of foods are best for you.

- **Practice stress management**: Stress can exacerbate physical symptoms and make them worse. Finding ways to manage stress, such as meditation, yoga, or deep breathing, can help you feel better and improve your overall well-being.

- **Seek support**: Navigating the physical challenges of breast cancer can be easier with the right support. Reach out to family and friends, join a support group, or talk to a counselor if you need someone to talk to.

- **Seek medical attention**: If you're experiencing pain or other symptoms that are affecting your quality of life, seek medical attention right away. Your healthcare team can provide treatment and support to help relieve your symptoms and improve your overall well-being.

- **Rest and relax**: Taking time to rest and relax can help you recharge and improve your overall well-being. Whether it's taking a nap, reading a book, or doing a relaxing activity, taking time to care for yourself is important.

Remember, everyone's experience with breast cancer is different, and what works for one person may not work for another. The important thing is to find what works for you and to reach out for help when you need it. With the right support and resources, you can navigate the physical challenges of breast cancer and maintain your quality of life.

Managing Pain and Discomfort

Breast cancer and its treatments can cause a range of physical symptoms, including pain and discomfort. Managing these symptoms is an important part of your care, as they can affect your quality of life and even your ability to complete your treatment. Here are some strategies for managing pain and discomfort:

1. **Talk to your healthcare team**: It's important to let your healthcare team know about any pain or discomfort you're experiencing. They can help you identify the cause of your symptoms and develop a plan to manage them.

2. **Use medication**: Pain medication is often the first line of defense for managing pain and discomfort. Your healthcare team can prescribe medication that's appropriate for your level of pain and your overall health.

3. **Use non-pharmacologic approaches**: There is a range of non-pharmacologic approaches to managing pain and discomfort. These may include relaxation techniques, such as deep breathing or meditation, physical therapy, or massage.

4. **Make lifestyle changes**: Making changes to your lifestyle can also help manage pain and discomfort. This may include getting enough rest, eating a healthy diet, and staying active, within your limits.

5. **Seek support**: Breast cancer and its treatments can be challenging both physically and emotionally. Seeking support from friends, family, or a support group can help you manage your symptoms and improve your overall well-being.

6. **Consider complementary therapies**: There is a range of complementary therapies that may help manage pain and discomfort, such as acupuncture, herbal supplements, or mind-body approaches. It's important to talk to your healthcare team before starting any complementary therapies, to ensure they're safe and effective for you.

7. **Participate in clinical trials**: Clinical trials are research studies that test new approaches to managing pain and other symptoms. By participating in a clinical trial, you may have access to new treatments that are not yet available to the general public.

Remember, managing pain and discomfort is an important part of your breast cancer care. It's important to talk to your healthcare team about any symptoms you're experiencing and work together to develop a plan to manage them. With the right support and resources, you can manage your symptoms and maintain your quality of life during and after treatment.

Maintaining a Healthy Lifestyle

Maintaining a healthy lifestyle is important for everyone, but it can be especially important for people who have been diagnosed with breast cancer. A healthy lifestyle can help you manage your symptoms, reduce your risk of cancer recurrence, and improve your overall well-being. Here are some strategies for maintaining a healthy lifestyle during and after breast cancer treatment:

1. **Eat a healthy diet**: Eating a healthy diet is important for managing your symptoms and improving your overall health. Aim for a diet that's high in fruits and vegetables, whole grains, and lean proteins. Avoid processed foods, sugary drinks, and foods that are high in saturated fats.

2. **Stay physically active**: Physical activity is important for managing your symptoms, reducing your risk of cancer recurrence, and improving your overall well-being. Aim for at least 30 minutes of moderate physical activity, such as walking, biking, or swimming, most days of the week.

3. **Maintain a healthy weight**: Maintaining a healthy weight is important for managing your symptoms and reducing your risk of cancer recurrence. If you're overweight or obese, talk to your healthcare team about ways to lose weight and maintain a healthy weight.

4. **Manage stress**: Stress can contribute to fatigue, anxiety, and other symptoms, so it's important to manage your stress levels. Try relaxation techniques, such as deep

breathing, meditation, or yoga, to help manage stress and improve your overall well-being.

5. **Limit alcohol consumption**: Drinking alcohol can increase your risk of cancer recurrence, so it's important to limit your alcohol consumption. If you do drink, limit your intake to one drink per day or less.

6. **Quit smoking**: Smoking can increase your risk of cancer recurrence, so it's important to quit smoking if you're a smoker. Talk to your healthcare team about resources to help you quit.

7. **Get regular check-ups**: Regular check-ups with your healthcare team are important for monitoring your symptoms, managing any side effects of treatment, and detecting any signs of cancer recurrence. Make sure to follow your healthcare team's recommendations for regular check-ups and screenings.

Remember, maintaining a healthy lifestyle is an important part of your breast cancer care. It's important to work with your healthcare team to develop a plan for maintaining a healthy lifestyle during and after treatment. With the right support and resources, you can manage your symptoms, reduce your risk of cancer recurrence, and improve your overall well-being.

CHAPTER 4

Moving Forward and Living Life to the Fullest

Moving forward and living life to the fullest after breast cancer treatment can be a complex and emotional process. It is important to remember that everyone's journey is unique and that there is no right or wrong way to move forward. Here are some strategies for moving forward and living life to the fullest after breast cancer treatment:

Set goals: Setting goals can help you stay focused and motivated as you move forward. Whether your goals are related to work, travel, hobbies, or personal relationships, it is important to set goals that are meaningful to you and that align with your values and priorities.

Stay connected: Staying connected with friends and loved ones is important for emotional support and for maintaining a sense of community. You can also consider joining a support group or connecting with other breast cancer survivors to share your experiences and find support.

Explore new interests: Exploring new interests can be a great way to discover new passions and reconnect with your sense of purpose. Whether it's taking up a new hobby, volunteering in your community, or pursuing a new career path, it is important to find activities that bring you joy and fulfillment.

Practice self-care: Practicing self-care is important for maintaining your physical and emotional well-being. This can include activities such as getting enough sleep, eating a healthy diet, engaging in regular physical activity, and practicing stress-reducing techniques such as meditation or yoga.

Celebrate your successes: Celebrating your successes, no matter how small, can help you stay motivated and positive as you move forward. Take time to acknowledge and celebrate your accomplishments, and don't be afraid to give yourself credit for your hard work and perseverance.

Talk to your healthcare team: Your healthcare team can provide valuable support and guidance as you move forward after breast cancer treatment. Be sure to stay in touch with your healthcare team and follow their recommendations for follow-up care and screenings.

Remember, moving forward and living life to the fullest after breast cancer treatment is a process, and it may take time to find your new sense of normalcy. Be kind to yourself and patient with the process, and don't be afraid to ask for help or support when you need it. With the right mindset, support, and resources, you can move forward with confidence and live a fulfilling and rewarding life after breast cancer.

Setting Goals and Priorities

Setting goals and priorities can be an important part of the breast cancer journey, especially when it comes to moving forward and adjusting to life after treatment. Here are some strategies for setting goals and priorities that can help you live a fulfilling and rewarding life after breast cancer:

Identify what's important to you: Start by identifying what's most important to you in life, whether it's spending time with family and friends, pursuing a hobby, traveling, or advancing your career. Think about what brings you joy and fulfillment, and make a list of your top priorities.

Make specific, measurable goals: Once you've identified you priorities, it's time to set specific, measurable goals that align with those priorities. For example, if one of your priorities is to spend more time with family and friends, you might set a goal to plan one social activity per week. Make sure your goals are specific, measurable, and realistic, and that you have a clear plan for achieving them.

Break goals down into smaller steps: Achieving big goals can be overwhelming, so it's important to break them down into smaller, manageable steps. For example, if your goal is to run a 5K race, you might break that goal down into smaller steps such as running for 20 minutes a day, increasing your running time by five minutes per week, and joining a local running club.

Use visual aids: Visual aids such as vision boards or daily reminders can help stay motivated and focused on your goals.

Create a vision board with images and words that inspire you, or set daily reminders on your phone to keep you on track.

Celebrate your successes: Celebrating your successes, no matter how small, can help keep you motivated and positive. When you achieve a goal, take time to acknowledge your hard work and give yourself credit for your accomplishment. Celebrate with a special activity or treat that aligns with your priorities and values.

Remember, setting goals and priorities is a personal process, and what works for one person may not work for another. Take the time to reflect on your values and priorities, and set goals that align with those values. With patience, persistence, and a clear plan, you can achieve your goals and live a fulfilling and rewarding life after breast cancer.

Finding Purpose and Meaning

Breast cancer is a life-altering experience that can cause a person to re-evaluate their priorities, goals, and values. For many, it can be a time of personal transformation and growth. Finding purpose and meaning after a breast cancer diagnosis can be a powerful way to cope with the challenges of the disease and find new ways to thrive. Here are some strategies for finding purpose and meaning after a breast cancer diagnosis:

1. **Reflect on your values**: Take time to reflect on your values and what is most important to you in life. Ask yourself what gives your life meaning and purpose. Identifying your values can help guide your decisions and

activities and can help you identify opportunities for personal growth and fulfillment.

2. **Engage in meaningful activities**: Engage in activities that align with your values and bring you joy. Whether it's volunteering for a cause you care about, pursuing a hobby, or spending time with loved ones, engaging in activities that make you feel fulfilled and happy can help you find meaning and purpose in your life.

3. **Find new opportunities for personal growth**: Breast cancer can be a time of personal growth and transformation. Take advantage of this time to reflect on your life and explore new avenues for personal growth and development. This might mean taking a course, learning a new skill, or exploring a new hobby.

4. **Focus on the positive**: While breast cancer can be a challenging experience, it can also bring unexpected blessings and positive changes. Focus on the positive aspects of your journey and look for opportunities to learn, grow, and give back.

5. **Connect with others**: Building connections with others who have been through similar experiences can be a powerful way to find purpose and meaning after breast cancer. Consider joining a support group, connecting with other survivors, or reaching out to others in your community who may be going through a similar experience.

6. **Find meaning in your breast cancer journey**: For some, finding meaning in their breast cancer journey can be a powerful way to cope with the disease. This might mean using your experience to help others going through a similar experience, becoming an advocate for breast cancer research, or simply finding a way to make sense of your diagnosis and treatment.

Remember, finding purpose and meaning is a personal process, and what works for one person may not work for another. Take the time to explore your values, engage in meaningful activities, and focus on the positive aspects of your journey. With patience, persistence, and a willingness to explore new opportunities, you can find purpose and meaning after breast cancer.

Building Resilience for the Future

Building resilience is an essential aspect of coping with the challenges of breast cancer and creating a positive future. Resilience refers to a person's ability to adapt to change, cope with adversity, and maintain a sense of purpose and meaning in life. Here are some strategies for building resilience for the future:

1. **Cultivate a positive mindset**: A positive mindset can help you face challenges with optimism and hope. Focus on your strengths, identify positive aspects of your life, and practice gratitude. Try to reframe negative thoughts into positive ones and focus on solutions rather than problems.

2. **Nurture a support system**: A support system can be a critical source of resilience. Reach out to loved ones, connect with a support group, or seek professional

counseling. Having a supportive network can help you stay motivated, maintain perspective, and navigate challenging times.

3. **Take care of yourself**: Self-care is essential for building resilience. Make time for regular exercise, healthy eating, and getting enough sleep. Manage stress through mindfulness practices, relaxation techniques, or other stress-reducing activities.

4. **Set achievable goals**: Setting achievable goals can help you maintain a sense of purpose and motivation. Identify small steps you can take toward achieving your goals and celebrate your progress along the way.

5. **Embrace change and uncertainty:** Change and uncertainty are a part of life. Learning to embrace them can help you build resilience. Focus on what you can control and take action where you can. Practice acceptance of what you can't control, and find ways to adapt and adjust to changing circumstances.

6. **Cultivate a sense of meaning and purpose**: A sense of meaning and purpose can help you find hope and motivation during difficult times. Reflect on your values and what gives your life meaning. Identify ways you can make a positive impact on the world and engage in activities that align with your values and purpose.

Remember, building resilience is a lifelong process. It requires effort, patience, and a willingness to learn from challenges and etbacks. By focusing on cultivating a positive mindset, nurturing a support system, taking care of yourself, setting achievable goals, embracing change and uncertainty, and cultivating a sense of meaning and purpose, you can build resilience that will help you navigate the challenges of breast cancer and beyond.

Celebrating Your Triumphs

Celebrating your triumphs is an important aspect of coping with breast cancer and moving forward in a positive direction. Breast cancer treatment can be a long and challenging journey, and it's essential to acknowledge and celebrate your accomplishments along the way. Here are some ways to celebrate your triumphs:

1. **Recognize your progress**: Celebrate the milestones you've achieved, no matter how small. Take time to reflect on the challenges you've overcome and the progress you've made. Write down your accomplishments and revisit them when you need a reminder of your strength and resilience.

2. **Treat yourself**: Do something special for yourself to mark your progress. This could be anything from a relaxing day at the spa to a special meal at your favorite restaurant. Treating yourself can help you feel proud of your achievements and remind you of the importance of self-care.

3. **Celebrate with loved ones**: Share your accomplishments with those closest to you. Celebrate with family and friends, host a dinner party, or plan a special outing. Sharing your triumphs with others can help you feel supported and surrounded by love.

4. **Volunteer and give back**: Volunteering and giving back can be a meaningful way to celebrate your triumphs. Consider volunteering for a breast cancer organization, supporting a friend who is going through a similar journey, or participating in a fundraising event. Giving back can help you feel empowered and give you a sense of purpose.

5. **Reflect on your journey**: Take time to reflect on your breast cancer journey and the lessons you've learned along the way. Think about the ways you've grown and the positive changes you've made in your life. Celebrating your triumphs can help you move forward with a renewed sense of purpose and optimism.

Remember, celebrating your triumphs is an ongoing process. Breast cancer can be a long and challenging journey, but taking time to acknowledge and celebrate your accomplishments can help you stay motivated and positive. By recognizing your progress, treating yourself, celebrating with loved ones, volunteering and giving back, and reflecting on your journey, you can celebrate your triumphs and move forward with confidence and optimism.

Looking Ahead with Hope and Confidence

Looking ahead with hope and confidence is an important part of the breast cancer journey. After completing treatment, many people feel a sense of relief and hope for the future. However, it's not uncommon to also feel anxious or uncertain about what lies ahead. Here are some ways to look ahead with hope and confidence:

1. **Focus on the positive**: Try to focus on the positive aspects of your life and the things that bring you joy. Think about the things you are grateful for and take time to appreciate the small things in life.

2. **Set goals**: Setting goals can help you stay focused and motivated. Think about the things you would like to achieve in the future and make a plan to work towards them. Whether it's learning a new skill or traveling to a new destination, setting goals can give you a sense of purpose and direction.

3. **Connect with others**: Staying connected with family, friends, and other breast cancer survivors can be an important source of support and encouragement. Join a support group, connect with others online, or attend local events and activities to meet others who have gone through similar experiences.

4. **Take care of yourself**: Taking care of your physical, emotional, and mental health is crucial to moving forward with hope and confidence. Exercise regularly, eat a healthy diet, get enough sleep, and make time for self-care activities that help you relax and recharge.

5. **Talk to your healthcare team**: Your healthcare team can provide guidance and support as you transition into life after treatment. Talk to your doctor about any concerns or questions you may have and work together to develop a plan for follow-up care.

6. **Embrace new opportunities**: Breast cancer can be a life-changing experience, but it can also open up new opportunities and experiences. Consider exploring new hobbies or interests, trying new things, and stepping outside of your comfort zone.

Remember, moving forward with hope and confidence is a journey, and it's important to be patient and kind to yourself as you navigate the ups and downs of life after breast cancer. By focusing on the positive, setting goals, connecting with others, taking care of yourself, talking to your healthcare team, and embracing new opportunities, you can move forward with hope and confidence and live your life to the fullest.

Final Thoughts and Encouragement.

Breast cancer can be a challenging journey, both physically and emotionally. However, with the right support and resources, it is possible to overcome the disease and move forward with a new appreciation for life.

It's essential to remember that you are not alone. There are many resources available, from medical professionals to support groups and online communities, that can provide guidance and encouragement throughout your journey. Remember to prioritize self-care and take time to focus on your mental and emotional well-being.

The road to recovery may not always be easy, but it's important to celebrate your victories along the way, no matter how small they may seem. Every step forward is a step in the right direction.

Most importantly, stay positive and keep looking ahead with hope and confidence. You are a survivor, and your journey can serve as an inspiration to others. By sharing your experiences and triumphs, you can help raise awareness and support for others who are facing similar challenges.

www.ingramcontent.com/pod-product-compliance
Lightning Source LLC
Chambersburg PA
CBHW061606250726
48657CB00017B/2185